Stick With It

Diet & Fitness Journal

ISBN: 978-1942156307

Majestic Publishing, LLC
PO Box 1560
Lithonia, GA 30058

www.majesticpublishing.net

Date: ____________ Weight: ____________

How I Feel: ____________ Goals: ____________

Nutrition

Meal	Decription	Calories	Fat	Protein	Carbs
Breakfast					
Lunch					
Snack					
Dinner					
TODAY'S TOTALS					

Fitness

Workout	Reps	Weight	Notes

Mind

How I Feel Today...

My Goals For Tomorrow...

Date: ______________________ Weight: ______________________

How I Feel: ______________________ Goals: ______________________

Nutrition

Meal	Decription	Calories	Fat	Protein	Carbs
Breakfast					
Lunch					
Snack					
Dinner					
TODAY'S TOTALS					

Fitness

Workout	Reps	Weight	Notes

Mind

How I Feel Today...

My Goals For Tomorrow...

Date: ______________________ Weight: ______________________

How I Feel: ______________________ Goals: ______________________

Nutrition

Meal	Decription	Calories	Fat	Protein	Carbs
Breakfast					
Lunch					
Snack					
Dinner					
	TODAY'S TOTALS				

Fitness

Workout	Reps	Weight	Notes

Mind

How I Feel Today...

My Goals For Tomorrow...

Date: ______________________ Weight: ______________________

How I Feel: ______________________ Goals: ______________________

Nutrition

Meal	Decription	Calories	Fat	Protein	Carbs
Breakfast					
Lunch					
Snack					
Dinner					
TODAY'S TOTALS					

Fitness

Workout	Reps	Weight	Notes

Mind

How I Feel Today...

My Goals For Tomorrow...

Date: ______________________ Weight: ______________________

How I Feel: ______________________ Goals: ______________________

Nutrition

Meal	Decription	Calories	Fat	Protein	Carbs
Breakfast					
Lunch					
Snack					
Dinner					
	TODAY'S TOTALS				

Fitness

Workout	Reps	Weight	Notes

Mind

How I Feel Today...

My Goals For Tomorrow...

Date: ______________________ Weight: ______________________

How I Feel: ______________________ Goals: ______________________

Nutrition

Meal	Decription	Calories	Fat	Protein	Carbs
Breakfast					
Lunch					
Snack					
Dinner					
	TODAY'S TOTALS				

Fitness

Workout	Reps	Weight	Notes

Mind

How I Feel Today...

My Goals For Tomorrow...

Date: ______________________ Weight: ______________________

How I Feel: ______________________ Goals: ______________________

Nutrition

Meal	Decription	Calories	Fat	Protein	Carbs
Breakfast					
Lunch					
Snack					
Dinner					
TODAY'S TOTALS					

Fitness

Workout	Reps	Weight	Notes

Mind

How I Feel Today...

My Goals For Tomorrow...

Date: ______________________ Weight: ______________________

How I Feel: ______________________ Goals: ______________________

Nutrition

Meal	Decription	Calories	Fat	Protein	Carbs
Breakfast					
Lunch					
Snack					
Dinner					
	TODAY'S TOTALS				

Fitness

Workout	Reps	Weight	Notes

Mind

How I Feel Today...

My Goals For Tomorrow...

Date:

Weight:

How I Feel:

Goals:

Nutrition

Meal	Decription	Calories	Fat	Protein	Carbs
Breakfast					
Lunch					
Snack					
Dinner					
TODAY'S TOTALS					

Fitness

Workout	Reps	Weight	Notes

Mind

How I Feel Today...

My Goals For Tomorrow...

Date: ______________________ Weight: ______________________

How I Feel: ______________________ Goals: ______________________

Nutrition

Meal	Decription	Calories	Fat	Protein	Carbs
Breakfast					
Lunch					
Snack					
Dinner					
TODAY'S TOTALS					

Fitness

Workout	Reps	Weight	Notes

Mind

How I Feel Today...

My Goals For Tomorrow...

Date: ____________________ Weight: ____________________

How I Feel: ____________________ Goals: ____________________

Nutrition

Meal	Decription	Calories	Fat	Protein	Carbs
Breakfast					
Lunch					
Snack					
Dinner					
	TODAY'S TOTALS				

Fitness

Workout	Reps	Weight	Notes

Mind

How I Feel Today...

My Goals For Tomorrow...

Date: ____________________ Weight: ____________________

How I Feel: ____________________ Goals: ____________________

Nutrition

Meal	Decription	Calories	Fat	Protein	Carbs
Breakfast					
Lunch					
Snack					
Dinner					
	TODAY'S TOTALS				

Fitness

Workout	Reps	Weight	Notes

Mind

How I Feel Today...

My Goals For Tomorrow...

Date: ____________________ Weight: ____________________

How I Feel: ____________________ Goals: ____________________

Nutrition

Meal	Decription	Calories	Fat	Protein	Carbs
Breakfast					
Lunch					
Snack					
Dinner					
TODAY'S TOTALS					

Fitness

Workout	Reps	Weight	Notes

Mind

How I Feel Today...

My Goals For Tomorrow...

Date: ____________________ Weight: ____________________

How I Feel: ____________________ Goals: ____________________

Nutrition

Meal	Decription	Calories	Fat	Protein	Carbs
Breakfast					
Lunch					
Snack					
Dinner					
TODAY'S TOTALS					

Fitness

Workout	Reps	Weight	Notes

Mind

How I Feel Today...

My Goals For Tomorrow...

Date: ______________________ Weight: ______________________

How I Feel: ______________________ Goals: ______________________

Nutrition

Meal	Decription	Calories	Fat	Protein	Carbs
Breakfast					
Lunch					
Snack					
Dinner					
	TODAY'S TOTALS				

Fitness

Workout	Reps	Weight	Notes

Mind

How I Feel Today...

My Goals For Tomorrow...

Date: ____________________ Weight: ____________________

How I Feel: ____________________ Goals: ____________________

Nutrition

Meal	Decription	Calories	Fat	Protein	Carbs
Breakfast					
Lunch					
Snack					
Dinner					
	TODAY'S TOTALS				

Fitness

Workout	Reps	Weight	Notes

Mind

How I Feel Today...

My Goals For Tomorrow...

Date: ______________________ Weight: ______________________

How I Feel: ______________________ Goals: ______________________

Nutrition

Meal	Decription	Calories	Fat	Protein	Carbs
Breakfast					
Lunch					
Snack					
Dinner					
TODAY'S TOTALS					

Fitness

Workout	Reps	Weight	Notes

Mind

How I Feel Today...

My Goals For Tomorrow...

Date: ______________________ Weight: ______________________

How I Feel: ______________________ Goals: ______________________

Nutrition

Meal	Decription	Calories	Fat	Protein	Carbs
Breakfast					
Lunch					
Snack					
Dinner					
TODAY'S TOTALS					

Fitness

Workout	Reps	Weight	Notes

Mind

How I Feel Today...

My Goals For Tomorrow...

Date: ____________________ Weight: ____________________

How I Feel: ____________________ Goals: ____________________

Nutrition

Meal	Decription	Calories	Fat	Protein	Carbs
Breakfast					
Lunch					
Snack					
Dinner					
TODAY'S TOTALS					

Fitness

Workout	Reps	Weight	Notes

Mind

How I Feel Today...

My Goals For Tomorrow...

Date: ______________________ Weight: ______________________

How I Feel: ______________________ Goals: ______________________

Nutrition

Meal	Decription	Calories	Fat	Protein	Carbs
Breakfast					
Lunch					
Snack					
Dinner					
	TODAY'S TOTALS				

Fitness

Workout	Reps	Weight	Notes

Mind

How I Feel Today...

My Goals For Tomorrow...

Date: ______________________ Weight: ______________________

How I Feel: ______________________ Goals: ______________________

Nutrition

Meal	Decription	Calories	Fat	Protein	Carbs
Breakfast					
Lunch					
Snack					
Dinner					
	TODAY'S TOTALS				

Fitness

Workout	Reps	Weight	Notes

Mind

How I Feel Today...

My Goals For Tomorrow...

Date: ______________________ Weight: ______________________

How I Feel: ______________________ Goals: ______________________

Nutrition

Meal	Decription	Calories	Fat	Protein	Carbs
Breakfast					
Lunch					
Snack					
Dinner					
TODAY'S TOTALS					

Fitness

Workout	Reps	Weight	Notes

Mind

How I Feel Today...

My Goals For Tomorrow...

Date: ______________________ Weight: ______________________

How I Feel: ______________________ Goals: ______________________

Nutrition

Meal	Decription	Calories	Fat	Protein	Carbs
Breakfast					
Lunch					
Snack					
Dinner					
	TODAY'S TOTALS				

Fitness

Workout	Reps	Weight	Notes

Mind

How I Feel Today...

My Goals For Tomorrow...

Date: ____________________ Weight: ____________________

How I Feel: ____________________ Goals: ____________________

Nutrition

Meal	Decription	Calories	Fat	Protein	Carbs
Breakfast					
Lunch					
Snack					
Dinner					
	TODAY'S TOTALS				

Fitness

Workout	Reps	Weight	Notes

Mind

How I Feel Today...

My Goals For Tomorrow...

Date: ______________________ Weight: ______________________

How I Feel: ______________________ Goals: ______________________

Nutrition

Meal	Decription	Calories	Fat	Protein	Carbs
Breakfast					
Lunch					
Snack					
Dinner					
	TODAY'S TOTALS				

Fitness

Workout	Reps	Weight	Notes

Mind

How I Feel Today...

My Goals For Tomorrow...

Date: ______________________ Weight: ______________________

How I Feel: ______________________ Goals: ______________________

Nutrition

Meal	Decription	Calories	Fat	Protein	Carbs
Breakfast					
Lunch					
Snack					
Dinner					
	TODAY'S TOTALS				

Fitness

Workout	Reps	Weight	Notes

Mind

How I Feel Today...

My Goals For Tomorrow...

Date: ______________________ Weight: ______________________

How I Feel: ______________________ Goals: ______________________

Nutrition

Meal	Decription	Calories	Fat	Protein	Carbs
Breakfast					
Lunch					
Snack					
Dinner					
TODAY'S TOTALS					

Fitness

Workout	Reps	Weight	Notes

Mind

How I Feel Today...

My Goals For Tomorrow...

Date: ______________________ Weight: ______________________

How I Feel: ______________________ Goals: ______________________

Nutrition

Meal	Decription	Calories	Fat	Protein	Carbs
Breakfast					
Lunch					
Snack					
Dinner					
	TODAY'S TOTALS				

Fitness

Workout	Reps	Weight	Notes

Mind

How I Feel Today...

My Goals For Tomorrow...

Date: ______________________ Weight: ______________________

How I Feel: ______________________ Goals: ______________________

Nutrition

Meal	Decription	Calories	Fat	Protein	Carbs
Breakfast					
Lunch					
Snack					
Dinner					
	TODAY'S TOTALS				

Fitness

Workout	Reps	Weight	Notes

Mind

How I Feel Today...

My Goals For Tomorrow...

Date: ____________________ Weight: ____________________

How I Feel: ____________________ Goals: ____________________

Nutrition

Meal	Decription	Calories	Fat	Protein	Carbs
Breakfast					
Lunch					
Snack					
Dinner					
	TODAY'S TOTALS				

Fitness

Workout	Reps	Weight	Notes

Mind

How I Feel Today...

My Goals For Tomorrow...

Date: ______________________ Weight: ______________________

How I Feel: ______________________ Goals: ______________________

Nutrition

Meal	Decription	Calories	Fat	Protein	Carbs
Breakfast					
Lunch					
Snack					
Dinner					
TODAY'S TOTALS					

Fitness

Workout	Reps	Weight	Notes

Mind

How I Feel Today...

My Goals For Tomorrow...

Date: ____________________ Weight: ____________________

How I Feel: ____________________ Goals: ____________________

Nutrition

Meal	Decription	Calories	Fat	Protein	Carbs
Breakfast					
Lunch					
Snack					
Dinner					
	TODAY'S TOTALS				

Fitness

Workout	Reps	Weight	Notes

Mind

How I Feel Today...

My Goals For Tomorrow...

Date: ______________________ Weight: ______________________

How I Feel: ______________________ Goals: ______________________

Nutrition

Meal	Decription	Calories	Fat	Protein	Carbs
Breakfast					
Lunch					
Snack					
Dinner					
TODAY'S TOTALS					

Fitness

Workout	Reps	Weight	Notes

Mind

How I Feel Today...

My Goals For Tomorrow...

Date: ______________________ Weight: ______________________

How I Feel: ______________________ Goals: ______________________

______________________ ______________________

______________________ ______________________

______________________ ______________________

Nutrition

Meal	Decription	Calories	Fat	Protein	Carbs
Breakfast					
Lunch					
Snack					
Dinner					
	TODAY'S TOTALS				

Fitness

Workout	Reps	Weight	Notes

Mind

How I Feel Today...

My Goals For Tomorrow...

Date: ______________________ Weight: ______________________

How I Feel: ______________________ Goals: ______________________

Nutrition

Meal	Decription	Calories	Fat	Protein	Carbs
Breakfast					
Lunch					
Snack					
Dinner					
	TODAY'S TOTALS				

Fitness

Workout	Reps	Weight	Notes

Mind

How I Feel Today...

My Goals For Tomorrow...

Date: ______________________ Weight: ______________________

How I Feel: ______________________ Goals: ______________________

Nutrition

Meal	Decription	Calories	Fat	Protein	Carbs
Breakfast					
Lunch					
Snack					
Dinner					
	TODAY'S TOTALS				

Fitness

Workout	Reps	Weight	Notes

Mind

How I Feel Today...

My Goals For Tomorrow...

Date: ____________ Weight: ____________

How I Feel: ____________ Goals: ____________

Nutrition

Meal	Decription	Calories	Fat	Protein	Carbs
Breakfast					
Lunch					
Snack					
Dinner					
TODAY'S TOTALS					

Fitness

Workout	Reps	Weight	Notes

Mind

How I Feel Today...

My Goals For Tomorrow...

Date: ______________________ Weight: ______________________

How I Feel: ______________________ Goals: ______________________

Nutrition

Meal	Decription	Calories	Fat	Protein	Carbs
Breakfast					
Lunch					
Snack					
Dinner					
	TODAY'S TOTALS				

Fitness

Workout	Reps	Weight	Notes

Mind

How I Feel Today...

My Goals For Tomorrow...

Date: ______________________ Weight: ______________________

How I Feel: ______________________ Goals: ______________________

Nutrition

Meal	Decription	Calories	Fat	Protein	Carbs
Breakfast					
Lunch					
Snack					
Dinner					
	TODAY'S TOTALS				

Fitness

Workout	Reps	Weight	Notes

Mind

How I Feel Today...

My Goals For Tomorrow...

Date: ______________________ Weight: ______________________

How I Feel: ______________________ Goals: ______________________

Nutrition

Meal	Decription	Calories	Fat	Protein	Carbs
Breakfast					
Lunch					
Snack					
Dinner					
	TODAY'S TOTALS				

Fitness

Workout	Reps	Weight	Notes

Mind

How I Feel Today...

My Goals For Tomorrow...

Date: ____________________ Weight: ____________________

How I Feel: ____________________ Goals: ____________________

Nutrition

Meal	Decription	Calories	Fat	Protein	Carbs
Breakfast					
Lunch					
Snack					
Dinner					
TODAY'S TOTALS					

Fitness

Workout	Reps	Weight	Notes

Mind

How I Feel Today...

My Goals For Tomorrow...

Date: ______________________ Weight: ______________________

How I Feel: ______________________ Goals: ______________________

Nutrition

Meal	Decription	Calories	Fat	Protein	Carbs
Breakfast					
Lunch					
Snack					
Dinner					
TODAY'S TOTALS					

Fitness

Workout	Reps	Weight	Notes

Mind

How I Feel Today...

My Goals For Tomorrow...

Date: ____________________ Weight: ____________________

How I Feel: ____________________ Goals: ____________________

Nutrition

Meal	Decription	Calories	Fat	Protein	Carbs
Breakfast					
Lunch					
Snack					
Dinner					
TODAY'S TOTALS					

Fitness

Workout	Reps	Weight	Notes

Mind

How I Feel Today...

My Goals For Tomorrow...

Date: ______________________ Weight: ______________________

How I Feel: ______________________ Goals: ______________________

Nutrition

Meal	Decription	Calories	Fat	Protein	Carbs
Breakfast					
Lunch					
Snack					
Dinner					
TODAY'S TOTALS					

Fitness

Workout	Reps	Weight	Notes

Mind

How I Feel Today...

My Goals For Tomorrow...

Date: ______________________ Weight: ______________________

How I Feel: ______________________ Goals: ______________________

Nutrition

Meal	Decription	Calories	Fat	Protein	Carbs
Breakfast					
Lunch					
Snack					
Dinner					
TODAY'S TOTALS					

Fitness

Workout	Reps	Weight	Notes

Mind

How I Feel Today...

My Goals For Tomorrow...

Date: ____________________ Weight: ____________________

How I Feel: ____________________ Goals: ____________________

Nutrition

Meal	Decription	Calories	Fat	Protein	Carbs
Breakfast					
Lunch					
Snack					
Dinner					
	TODAY'S TOTALS				

Fitness

Workout	Reps	Weight	Notes

Mind

How I Feel Today...

My Goals For Tomorrow...

Date: ____________________ Weight: ____________________

How I Feel: ____________________ Goals: ____________________

Nutrition

Meal	Decription	Calories	Fat	Protein	Carbs
Breakfast					
Lunch					
Snack					
Dinner					
TODAY'S TOTALS					

Fitness

Workout	Reps	Weight	Notes

Mind

How I Feel Today...

My Goals For Tomorrow...

Date: ______________________ Weight: ______________________

How I Feel: ______________________ Goals: ______________________

Nutrition

Meal	Decription	Calories	Fat	Protein	Carbs
Breakfast					
Lunch					
Snack					
Dinner					
	TODAY'S TOTALS				

Fitness

Workout	Reps	Weight	Notes

Mind

How I Feel Today...

My Goals For Tomorrow...

Date: ______________________ Weight: ______________________

How I Feel: ______________________ Goals: ______________________

Nutrition

Meal	Decription	Calories	Fat	Protein	Carbs
Breakfast					
Lunch					
Snack					
Dinner					
	TODAY'S TOTALS				

Fitness

Workout	Reps	Weight	Notes

Mind

How I Feel Today...

My Goals For Tomorrow...

Date: ______________________ Weight: ______________________

How I Feel: ______________________ Goals: ______________________

Nutrition

Meal	Decription	Calories	Fat	Protein	Carbs
Breakfast					
Lunch					
Snack					
Dinner					
	TODAY'S TOTALS				

Fitness

Workout	Reps	Weight	Notes

Mind

How I Feel Today...

My Goals For Tomorrow...

Date: ____________________ Weight: ____________________

How I Feel: ____________________ Goals: ____________________

Nutrition

Meal	Decription	Calories	Fat	Protein	Carbs
Breakfast					
Lunch					
Snack					
Dinner					
	TODAY'S TOTALS				

Fitness

Workout	Reps	Weight	Notes

Mind

How I Feel Today...

My Goals For Tomorrow...

Date: ______________________ Weight: ______________________

How I Feel: ______________________ Goals: ______________________

Nutrition

Meal	Decription	Calories	Fat	Protein	Carbs
Breakfast					
Lunch					
Snack					
Dinner					
	TODAY'S TOTALS				

Fitness

Workout	Reps	Weight	Notes

Mind

How I Feel Today...

My Goals For Tomorrow...

Made in the USA
Monee, IL
06 November 2026

67375724R00059